I0440870

Sugar Addiction –
Beat Sugar Addiction Today

Tina Johnson

Copyright © 2013 Tina Johnson

All rights reserved.

ISBN: ISBN-10:1490908358
ISBN- ISBN-13:978-1490908359
:

DEDICATED TO YOU

This is what people don't understand: obesity is a symptom of poverty. It's not a lifestyle choice where people are just eating and not exercising. It's because kids - and this is the problem with school lunch right now - are getting sugar, fat, empty calories - lots of calories - but no nutrition.

Tom Colicchio

Sugar is more present in America or England than it is in France. I think there is an addiction to sweetness.

Pierre Dukan

CONTENTS

INTRODUCTION

Sugar addiction is generally thought of as a person having a sweet tooth, or sugar craving, but the reality is that sugar can be extremely addictive. One of the main problems with our traditional western diet is that sugar is almost everywhere and in numerous foodstuffs, making it almost impossible for people who have a sugar addiction to avoid. Whilst sugar addiction isn't regarded as an actual physical addiction it does seem to have a link to an emotional dependence.

The idea of a "Sugar Addiction" was initially popularized by Kathleen DesMaisons, PhD, an authority in the psychology of addiction. She explained it as being a measurable occurrence brought on by triggering receptors in the brain. Other studies have established that sugar can work as a painkiller, and that sugar's side effects can be obstructed with the very same drug treatments that obstruct the effects of morphine. Whilst sugar craving is yet to have been given its name formally many studies show that sugar is indeed addictive, bring about all manner of health problems that come about when too much sugar enters into our diet like diabetes, obesity, hyperactivity etc. While only until recently this addiction had been overlooked new research has identified just how widespread and severe this problem really is.

The notion that a sugar addiction is actually a real world and measurable thing came about recently when scientists at Princeton University made it possible to display sugar addiction in rats. In their study they withheld food items from the rats for around 4 hours after waking (equal to missing out on breakfast) after which they fed the rats' normal food plus some sugar water along with it. After some time, the rats began to quickly run to the sugared water, in some cases "bingeing" on it, and often drinking it in the first hour. Finally when the sweetened water was finally taken away, the lab rats showed the normal typical signs and symptoms of sugar withdrawal: teeth chattering and shaking. And whenever the sugar was taken away, the researchers also found that there were changes in the animals' brain chemistry.

Having a sugar addiction can be hard to diagnose in that sometimes it may not seem to have any immediate effect on you. While it may cause headaches, feelings of "bloatedness" it can show up as other symptoms in other people. But in the end whatever symptoms it shows it usually leads to weight gain, which then brings about its own type of problems. Plus when you try to keep it out of your diet it causes you to crave it even more than before. In some cases you may end up going to your local store unconsciously buying that milk chocolate bar you said you've never touch again, and then you probably reason with yourself that it this is going to be the last time. Next time you'll walk straight past it and won't ever consider buy it again?

But surely sugar couldn't be all the dangerous could it...

DANGERS OF SUGAR

Due to our western diet most of us are eating more sugar than we ever have before and unfortunately this isn't something that going to stop anytime soon. So how did we get ourselves into this situation? It seems that there's a link between our high consumption of sugar and the growth of mass food production in the western world. We're now in the grips of a business whose aim is to create bigger profits rather than worrying about the health of the public.

If you're one of those people who finds it hard to avoid sugar you're not alone. Sugar addiction is so commonplace that most of us aren't aware just how much sugar has a hold over us, until we try to give it up. Eating sugary foods causes our bodies to stimulate the release of dopamine in the brain, which causes feelings of pleasure. Since we all like the feeling of pleasure it's understandable that we'd look for places where we can get more of it, even if it comes from a sugar bowl. This leads to a vicious cycle of our bodies turning to sugar more and more to boost those pleasurable feelings.

Consuming sugar in high quantities on a daily basis affects our bodies in various ways. Recent studies have linked sugar with disabling diseases such as kidney damage, cancer, a lower immune system and even heart disease. Apart from the physical effects sugar has on our body, it also causes emotional problems as well. Eating sugar in excessive quantities leads to high blood sugar spikes and the lows of this can cause anxiety, light headiness and irritability.

Sugar itself doesn't have the ability to get into the cells of our body and needs a key to get in and this is provided by the body in the form of insulin. Insulin is produced by the body in response to high blood sugar levels in the body. While this works well as "Mother Nature" intended the problems start when the body has to produce higher and higher quantities of insulin to cope with the higher and higher quantities of sugar. Our bodies can cope initially with these cycles but over time our pancreas can't keep up with the demands placed on it. This then eventually leads to insulin resistance and diabetes.

Excessive insulin production can lead to our bodies suffering from sugar lows which we can see the symptoms as memory failure, fatigue and tiredness, depression, anxiety and even rapid heartbeats. While this list of conditions may sound like something someone in a nursing home would be suffering from, more and more young people are exhibiting these conditions.

Sugar can also change the make of our blood chemistry so much so, that even just 2 spoons of sugar has an effect on the micro nutrients in it and throw our bodies blood chemistry out of whack. Our bodies are so finally tuned that too much sugar can affect the delicate levels of minerals causing levels to increase and others to decrease. Crucial minerals like phosphorus, magnesium, zinc and iron are very important to the body and even a lack of one of these elements can affect our body's functions.

Following on from how sugar affects our blood chemistry arthritis is another condition that some researchers believe is linked to our high sugar consumption. While arthritis is seen is another age related condition it's become more common place in younger people. Sugar due to its effects on mineral levels may also have a hand in this. As I wrote earlier a deficiency balance or mineral lack can have an effect on our joints where a build-up of toxic minerals including a calcium ends up causing spurs and other bone related problems.

If all this isn't enough to make you want to quit sugar I don't know what will. But for those of you that still want to kick sugar to the curb, its best to know your enemy. So what can you expect to feel when you come off sugar....?

SUGAR WITHDRAWAL – WHAT TO EXPECT WHEN YOU'RE COMING OFF SUGAR

As you'd expect coming off sugar does cause emotional swings. In a way it does make sense as sugar does have an effect on the chemicals in the brain, some would say even as closely as heroin addiction. When you withdraw from sugar your body will go through a re-balancing stage where you may feel more depressed and anxious but stick to your guns and this will pass. Another thing to point out that even if your blood sugar is returning to a normal level you may still feel low until your body readjusts to things.

So what can you expect to go through when going through sugar withdrawal?

Feeling Down Or Sad – As previously written coming off sugar causes a lot of moods swings and this may be something you notice the most. Don't be surprised if you're more irritable or short tempered than normal and even depressed. If you're already suffering from any type of depression this should be watched and taken account of while going through a sugar withdrawal. But having said that some people who've suffered from depression found that they didn't feel as depressed when they came off sugar.

Headaches And Fogginess In Your Thinking – Headaches are also a common complaint when going through a sugar withdrawal. Like feeling sad or down this is probably down to a change in the brains chemistry or a change in stress levels. Some people also complain of a general feeling of fogginess in their thinking or keeping concentration. These should pass in a matter of days but if they continue longer than expected a visit to your doctor may be in order to find the cause of the problem.

Fatigue – In our busy lives we're constantly looking for ways to boost our energy levels, so don't be surprised if you've been using sugar like this. This may take a few days to spring back from but if you're eating healthier and keeping away from sugar your body and adrenal glands will get things back under control again.

Sleep - As well as feeling tired all the time you may notice some changes at bedtime. This is a natural thing and is your body detoxing and getting rid of sugar from your body. This should pass but if you're having problems, again have a chat with your doctor for advice.

More Sugar Cravings – Eating sugar has been a lifetime habit so don't be surprised if you start craving sugar more than ever at this time. In a way it's like when you're told you can't have something anymore (for example chocolate) you then want it even more so. Falling for these sugar craving now will only lengthen the withdrawal process and take you longer to quit. Stand your ground and they'll soon disappear.

When going through sugar withdrawal it's important to give your body the healthy foods it need to get through the detox process. There's no point in detoxing from sugar only to replace your addiction to sugar with some other artificial stimulant. Another point is to reduce salt and dairy intake while going through your detox as these have been found by some people cause a sweet craving. To get through the process try consuming small portion of protein throughout the day to soothe your craving. You can also use some herbal teas to keep yourself hydrated and help with the detox, fennel, nettle and liquorice can be helpful around this time.

Another things to be aware of when kicking the sugar habit is if soda or energy drinks were a major part of your diet you can suffer a caffeine withdrawal problem also. This is something you'll need to consider if you want to get rid of both at the same time try to also keep caffeine out of your diet. If you want to keep caffeine in your diet continue to do so but try to find a sugar free/dairy free way by drinking it black.

NATURAL SUGAR ALTERNATIVES

Using a natural alternatives to sugar could be just what you need to kick your sugar habit. You might think that because you've given up sugar you have to give up the sweet taste but this isn't so. With so many natural sweeteners on the market nowadays it's possible to soothe a sweet tooth without damaging your health.

Natural sugar alternatives can be found in all places from health food stores to your local supermarket. The benefit of these sweeteners is that they don't cause a large spike in the body's insulin levels that sugar does. This stops your body becoming insulin resistant and takes a lot of the strain off your pancreas. Natural sweeteners unlike sugar are unrefined meaning they have trace minerals still inside which your body can use. But a word of warning though natural sweeteners are still sugar and should be treated as such and should be eaten in moderation.

So what sugar alternatives are available…?

Agave – Agave is a natural sugar alternative that comes from the blue agave plant of Mexico. Like honey (raw version) agave has a low glycemic index meaning it doesn't cause wild fluctuations in blood sugar which makes it ideal for anyone suffering from diabetes. But while it is a healthier alternative to sugar it should be taken in moderation as it contains 960 calories per cup (much higher than sugar), which is something you should be aware of if you're also trying to lose weight. When buying agave try to find one that hasn't been overly processed as can lead to a far inferior product than the natural plant it came from.

Honey – One of the best natural sweeteners on the market is simply just plain old honey. It has a great taste doesn't have any chemicals or additives and contains trace amounts of B vitamins. While the only problem with honey is it comes in a sticky liquid form it has a long shelf life it's any easy way to sweeten up drinks and can be used in baking and cooking.

Maple Syrup – Pure maple syrup is made from sap from the maple tree. Apart from its sweetness maple syrup contains high levels of magnesium and zinc which helps our body's immune system. Maple syrup is also contains antioxidants, B vitamins and is rich in calcium. If used in moderation maple syrup can be a healthy alternative to sugar and is also suitable for a low carb diet programme.

Coconut Sugar (Coconut Palm Sugar) – Coconut sugar comes by various names including coconut palm sugar, coco sap sugar or coco sugar. This type of sugar has been around for thousands of years in South and South East Asia. Coconut sugar is produced by tapping coconut trees (just like maple trees) to draw out the sap. Coconut sugar is a healthy alternative to sugar for its low glycemic index and comes packed with minerals and amino acids. It also contain high levels of B vitamins, potassium, iron, zinc, potassium and inositol. Inostial is especially abundant and very helpful to the body for its impact on the nervous system and for creating healthy cells.

Xylitol – Xylitol is a white sweet substance that tastes and feels like normal sugar and can be used just like it, in drinks and home baking. Xylitol is found in the fibers of fruits and vegetables and is even naturally produced in small quantities in the body. It contains fewer calories and carbohydrates than normal sugar and rather than giving an instant boost of energy, it releases its energy as a slow trickle so you don't go through the high and lows of blood sugar levels. Xylitol also contains dietary fiber which helps with digestion, while most adults can get away with eating 40 grams of Xylitol it can cause diarrhoea in higher quantities.

Molasses – Molasses isn't a new sweetener but has been around a long time until refined white sugar took its place on the shopping aisles. Molasses was originally taken to the US continent by the early pilgrims that landed there. It's created by extracting the sugar from sugar beets and sugarcane. Once extracted the liquid is boiled up to three times to concentrate it, the first is called "Barbados" is the lightest in light and sweet, the second "Dark Molasses" is thicker and not as sweet and the third boiling is called "Blackstrap" and is the heartiest form of molasses. This form is also a lot sweeter than normal sugar so you'll require less to get the same sweetness.

Fruit juice – Fruit juice is a natural form of sugar and comes in deferring strengths and flavours. While you mightn't want to add apple or orange juice to any of your hot drinks it can be used successfully in cooking and baking. Fruit juice is best used in its freshest condition rather than in a concentrate form.

Brown Rice Syrup – Brown rice syrup is created by fermenting cooked brown rice. It's usually in a thick syrup state, brown in colour and has a hint of butter and caramel. It's about half as sweet as honey and although highly refined doesn't have the properties of white refined sugar. Due to its slower absorption by the body its energy is released over a longer period of time so you don't have the high peaks of white sugar. But although it has good qualities it's a high calorie sweetener and can add to weight gain if used in large quantities.

Tina Johnson

IS SALT TO BLAME FOR YOUR SUGAR CRAVINGS

Do you feel compelled to add an extra pinch of salt to your foods even before you taste them, chances are you've got an addiction to salt. But rather than adding salt to food for the added spice it gives to your food, you're probably adding it to because it puts you in a better mood. Something you've probably never thought of before?

According to researchers in the University of Iowa people who go without salt can become depressed, they found that salt puts people in as better mood and creates cravings comparable to a drug addiction.
Although some salt is needed in the body to help fluids pass through the body too much can cause health problems like high blood pressure and heart disease.

Professor Kim Johnson who did tests on rats found that when salt levels were lowered they lost that pleasure in things like a sugary drink. They also noticed a similar change in brain activity when the rats were denied drugs. "This suggests that salt need and cravings may be linked to the same brain pathways as those related to drug addiction and abuse," Prof Johnson said.

While some people out there may say that obesity is a matter of poor willpower it seems that manufacturers of food are designing food to become more addictive and salt seems to be a great way of doing this. While we all know the dangers of eating too much sugary foods but salt hasn't gotten as much press until lately, with ads on British TV highlighting the fact of high salt content in foods.

So now you need to become more aware of this because salt is now being added to almost all types of food and camouflaged with high levels of sugar to sweeten the taste. This is probably why a portion of salty French fries tastes so good when it's washed down with your favorite soda drink. The salt give us an initial hit and heightens the feeling for the sugary taste of the soda.

If you think about it we've allowed our food to dictate to us what we should eat rather than the other way around. So the next time you get a craving for something sweet think back, was that last food that I ate high in salt content? Chances are it was, and know you know where that sugar/food craving is coming from.

38 WAYS TO REDUCE YOUR SUGAR CRAVINGS

Did you know the average American goes through a whopping 160lbs of sugar per year. While you might know its obvious hiding places it's never far from our mouths. It can be found in less obvious places like ketchup, frozen peas, canned fruit and even some medicines. By learning to stop and control this menace you'll help free yourself up from the health problems it creates like obesity, heart disease and diabetes.

But don't think it's going to be easy like any drug addiction (some experts would put giving quitting sugar on the same scale as quitting smoking) your body will fight you along the way. Don't be surprised if you suffer from mood swings, irritability and feeling generally down when you try to kick the habit. But get through to the other side and your body will thank you for it by losing weight, increasing energy and being able to think clear headed.

So what that in mind let's get started on your path to quitting sugar...

Tip 1 - Apple Cider Vinegar - Try using some apple cider vinegar the next time you feel a sugar craving coming on. Make a mixture of 2 teaspoons to a glass of water and drink it down. Your caving should pass in less than 5 minutes.

Tip 2 - Never Shop on an Empty Stomach - Rather than just focusing on killing the sugar craving, try to limit how much you take into your home. So, never shop on an empty stomach. You'll have a tendency to fill up on more convenience and sugary foods if you've got an empty stomach.

Tip 3 - Lower Your Carbohydrates Intake - Most of us already eat enough carbs in our diet, your waistlines probably being trying to tell you this for a while. Lower your carbs and take in a high amount of protein in your daily diet. This will help to keep hunger at bay and help lower your sugar cravings.

Tip 4 - Are You Suffering From Candida? - Candida is a form of yeast that needs sugar to survive. Normally the bad bacteria in our gut are balanced out by the good bacteria, but taking in too much sugar upsets the balance and this becomes a breeding ground for Candida. If you're suffering from sugar cravings even though you shouldn't be hungry it's probably Candida causing the problem.

Tip 5 - Drink More Water - You may be misreading the signals from your stomach and confusing dehydration with a need for sugar. Try to get your recommended daily allowance of water and see if the feelings for sugar reduces.

Tip 5 - Reduce Your Tea and Coffee Use - Too much coffee and tea can cause dehydration and also a drop in blood sugar levels. This drop then causes feelings of hunger and a need for sugar. Try to swap your tea drinking for more herbal teas like green tea which is great for balancing blood sugar levels.

Tip 7 - Is It Sugar or Emotional? - Is your need for sugar linked to a physical problem or an emotional problem? Are you using sugar as an emotional band aid to cover up something else? E.F.T (or tapping) is an excellent way to uncover and clear sugar cravings and problems you may have with food. Visit YouTube.com for lots of E.F.T related videos that will help you uncover and clear your problem.

Tip 8 - Brush Your Teeth after You Eat - Brushing our teeth after a meal is a signal to our brain that feeding time is over. By cleaning our teeth with a fresh "minty" tooth paste it gives a feeling of cleanness which may make you less likely to grab something sweet.

Tip 9 - Don't Skip Breakfast - Having a good breakfast that includes some type of protein helps prevent those sugar drops and visits to the vending machine latter in the morning. Research done in a US university found that having breakfast that was higher in protein had an effect on hunger levels for the rest of the day. Even something as simple as having a boiled egg made a big difference.

Tip 10 - Do Snack Swap - If your snacks come in a wrapper they're probably going to do nothing to help reduce your sugar cravings. Try to substitute fruit and healthy snacks for sugary ones and the healthy complex carbohydrates will reduce your sugar cravings and give the body the fuel and energy it really needs.

Tip 11 - Stay Away From White Foods - *"If it's white it not alright!"* should be your new motto. Foods that are white like pasta, white bread and white rice, are big culprits for causing major sugar spikes and crashes. Stick to the brown versions of bread, pasta and rice and you'll start to notice your sugar levels stay on a more balanced level. Whole foods are basically unprocessed foods - wholemeal bread with grains, fruit, vegetables, meat, fish, eggs, cheese, nuts and pulses.

Tip 12 - Slow Down Your Eating - Do you eat too fast? Did you know that it takes your brain at least 20 minutes to realize that it's full? Slow down your eating and really taste your food as you're eating it and you'll help your body to better digest and absorb the nutrients and stop sugar cravings.

Tip 13 - Keep A Food Journal – Keeping a food journal can be a great way to take note of all that unconscious eating that we do through your day. A bit of chocolate here, a can of coke there and we never notice it. But by keeping a journal (even for a week) you'll start to take note of how you're eating and what foods are causing your sugar cravings.

Tip 14 – Top Up On Your Vitamins – Low levels of Vitamins such as Zinc, Chromium, Manganese, Magnesium can be the cause behind your sugar cravings. Having zinc deficiency can result in low insulin levels, which can lead to a craving for sugar and low chromium levels makes it harder for insulin to efficiently remove sugar from the blood. Try to increase your intake of these important minerals with supplements or through your diet. Foods such as beef, pork, chickpeas, almonds and oatmeal all contain Zinc.

Tip 15 – Get A Medical Check – If your sugar cravings are out of control, a possible visit to your doctor for some blood work could be in order. Those sugar cravings could be the onset of some type or condition that you'll need to have looked at.

Tip 16 – Drink More Milk – A low intake of milk or rather having low levels of calcium can be a cause of sugar cravings. The protein in milk also helps to keep your hunger at bay.

Tip 17 – Distract Yourself – Try not to think of a pink elephant and all you can think of is a pink elephant. Try not to think about that craving you have for sugar and you're bound to keep thinking about it. Try to find ways to distract yourself from the thoughts of food by going for a walk, reading a book, playing around with that app on your iPhone. You'll be surprised that it you distract yourself for 5 -10 minutes the craving will pass.

Tip 18 – Leave Sugar at the Store – Try going cold turkey and keep all sugar containing foods out of your home. If you can't get your hands on it, you can't eat it. It will be hard not having them at hand when your craving strikes, but overtime they will reduce and won't be as strong any more. Keep fruit at hand as a healthy substitute.

Tip 19 – Eat More – If you find cravings come frequently between meal times break your eating routine from 3 to 5 meals per day. By eating more often you help to get blood sugar levels on an even keel and avoid the sugar craving dips. Also add more fibre containing foods helps to keep your stomach full for longer.

Tip 20 – Try Natural Ways To Lift Your Mood – Serotonin is a chemical that s released in the brain to make us feel happy and content. If we don't feel good about ourselves we usually go for something sugary to give us the same type of high. If you're feeling down try to find some natural ways to build up your serotonin levels, There are various ways you can do this including listening to your favorite music, any/or form of exercise that increases serotonin levels.

Tip 21 – Watch out for Artificial Sweeteners - Many people think that all they have to do is substitute artificial sweeteners for sugar to reduce their sugar cravings but it doesn't work. While using artificial sweeteners can help stem the tide it doesn't reduce the bad health effects of eating too much sugar. And some research indicates that artificial sweeteners may actually increase sugar cravings. Try removing them also from your diet and see if it helps you.

Tip 22 – Chew Gum – Chewing gum can be a great distraction method for sugar cravings. The craving doesn't seem as strong because your body is fooled with the chewing and it gives you a chance to distract your mouth until the sugar urge passes. Try to carry a piece of gum on you at all times so when you feel the need for something sweet you can keep it at bay.

Tip 23 - Reduce Stress – Cortisol is a hormone produced by the body during stressful times. This increase then leads to high blood sugar and sugar cravings. We also tend to look for sugary comforting foods in times of stress and the cycle continues around and around. Try to find natural ways to reduce stress levels such as Tai Chi, yoga, or meditation. Lower stress levels before meals also helps your body's digestion and absorption of nutrients. Also try to increase your intake of vitamin C as it's important for the production of the hormone cortisol. Similar to B complex vitamins, cortisol helps keep blood sugar stable during stress. As a result, vitamin C decreases the symptoms of low blood sugar and reduces sugar cravings.

Tip 24 – Up Your Intake of Omega 3 - Omega-3 fatty acids do a lot of important tasks in the body one of which is to elevate our mood by increasing natural presence of serotonin in the brain. Having natural high serotonin levels makes us less dependent on sugar to help stimulate our feel good factor. Serotonin also helps to regulate our appetite. Keeping it in check will help you stay full and, as a result diminish your sugar cravings. To get more omega 3 fatty acids in your diet you can either use omega 3 supplements or by eating more omega 3 foods like oily fish and flax oil,

Tip 25 - Get More Sleep – Not getting a good night's sleep can be bad for you both mentally and physically. Lack of sleep reduces the body's levels of leptin, which makes you crave carbohydrates. Also, going without sleep interrupts our body's ability to use carbohydrates properly. This then causes higher levels of glucose in your body, which then produces higher levels of insulin levels and more thus more fat storage on your body. The mental side of losing out on a good night's sleep is higher stress and cortisol levels, this increase in cortisol then increases our hunger levels.

Tip 26 – Add Cinnamon to Your Food – Cinnamon is an easy and healthy way to reduce blood sugar levels and the natural production of insulin. Sprinkle it sparingly (one quarter tea spoon is enough) on to morning cereals, breads and cakes.

Tip 27 – Ginseng – Ginseng helps the body to cope with stress without affecting your sleep, mood or appetite. Ginseng works on our nervous system by helping to increase energy levels, lower blood sugar levels and reduce sugar addiction. If you're the type of person who suffers from emotional eating due to stress this supplement can help to reduce this problem. But be warned that the effects can take up to 2 -3 months before you'll see its effects.

Tip 28 – Green Tea – Green tea has become very popular in the west due to the many health benefits it brings. Green tea has been found to improve our body's metabolism (so we burn more fat) and also help control our bodies blood sugar levels. There are no known side effects and it can be an easy easily used instead of coffee and black tea.

Tip 29 – Eat More Apples and Pears – Apples and pears are a great way to snack healthily and reduce sugar cravings. The pectin and soluble fiber found in apples and pears decreases blood-sugar levels, helping you avoid between-meal snacking. An added way to improve on the flavour and sugar craving power of each is to sprinkle them with cinnamon before eating.

Tip 30 – Add More Fat To Your Food – When the next sugar craving attacks try adding some extra extra coconut oil, mayonnaise or butter to your food. While it may sound a little weird some people swear it helps them through their sugar craving without eating unhealthy foods.

Tip 31 - L-Glutamine- Try taking 500 mg of l-glutamine prior to meals to help to curb sugar cravings. L- Glutamine as well as improving brain function also works as an added source of fuel for the digestive system. Just like having a healthy brain, a healthy digestive system will keep you from craving sugary food. L-Glutamine is available in most health food shops in either powdered or capsule form.

Tip 32 – Improve Your Breathing – One of the lesser known ways to reducing sugar cravings is by taking a few deep breaths. Breathing deeply and properly helps to get more oxygen into our blood stream and helps our bodies to process food better. Surprisingly the majority of us don't breathe properly any-more, we breathe only with the upper (smaller) portions of our lungs rather than the lower (larger) portion. By learning to breathe properly again you help your brain to function more clearly and not have to look to sugar for help. Proper breathing also helps to reduce stress levels which also helps with food cravings.

Tip 33 – Eat More Soy Products – Obesity and overeating have been found to be linked to low dopamine levels. When we feel high feelings of satisfaction and pleasure that's the work of dopamine. One way to improve the release of dopamine is by consuming more soy products. Soya also has the added benefits of being very good at levelling insulin levels and thus decreasing fat storage. This means that we convert less calories into fat from food that we eat.

Tip 34 – Stevia – Stevia a herb from South America used specifically to treat diabetes, due to the effect it has on lowering blood sugar levels. It contains no calories but has a taste that's hundreds of times higher than sugar. Unlike other sweeteners on the market which have the opposite effect Stevia helps with insulin levels and helps to lower blood glucose levels.

Tip 35 – Grapefruit – In research it was found that eating half a grapefruit before a meal or drinking a serving of grapefruit juice three times a day helped people drop more than three pounds in 12 weeks. The power of grapefruit lies in its phytochemicals which help to reduce insulin levels and forcing your body to convert calories into energy rather than fat.

Tip 36 – Flaxseed – Flaxseed is packed with protein and fiber and can help to provide bulk to your meals. Flaxseed has the ability to swell up to five times in size to provide giving a more feeling of lasting fullness after mealtime. Flax seed also stabilizes blood sugar levels help to reduces cravings,

Tip 37 – Licorice – Is a natural herb that's been used for centuries for both cooking and medicine purposes. It's a natural way to satisfy sugar cravings and increase energy levels. Licorice doesn't increase blood glucose levels when used and can be used as a sugar substitute. Most health food stores have in various forms from liquid to powder.

Tip 38 - And finally, all it takes is one sugary drink or food to trigger a sugar binge. To break your sugar cravings you'll need to begin by breaking your current eating habits. Have healthy snacks at hand and a meal plan will go a long way in preventing you from snacking both out of habit or from low blood sugar.

FINAL THOUGHTS

I want to congratulate you for purchasing this book but also for having the courage to kick sugar from your diet. I've done it myself and found that my life is so much better for having done so, my skin, energy levels and mood are so much improved so much when I gave sugar up.

But while you may be psyched up and ready to change your health once and for all there will be times when you may fall off the sugar free wagon. With that in mind I've put together a list of sugar facts that you can print off or keep close to hand to remind you of the dangers of refined sugar.

-Sugar can cause damage to your pancreas and has been linked to pancreatic cancer by researchers in Sweden. In some cases it raised cancer levels by 70%.
-Sugar suppresses your immune system which leaves you open to disease and infections. People who consume high levels of sugar have low levels of Vitamin C, A and B-12, and low levels of the mineral magnesium, iron, phosphorus and calcium.
-Sugar promotes inflammation and promotes disease and aging.
-Sugar can cause food allergies, high blood pressure, acne, eye problems, constipation, depression and headaches.
-Sugar is very closely linked to the close effects of drug abuse, for the feelings, cravings and withdrawal effects it causes. It's also as addictive as heroin and cocaine.
-Sugar can make you age faster, as it binds to the proteins to collagen and elastin in the skin breaking down its youthful and firm appearance.

If this short list isn't enough to want to make you quit sugar forever I don't what will?

Want to know what other readers thought of this book or want to leave me a comment? I'd love to read your thoughts on this book, if you could please take a moment now to leave me a comment on the book what you enjoyed or wanted more of, it will help me greatly in writing a better book for you.

Here's to your success and thanks in advance for your comments

Lots of love Tina!

RECOMMENDED READING

While I might feel I've written a great book I know there are some other great books that will also help you greatly. So with that in mind here are three other books I feel may be also be a great help to you.

Overcoming Sugar Addiction: How I Kicked My Sugar Habit and Created a Joyful Sugar Free Life.
http://www.amazon.com/Overcoming-Sugar-Addiction-Created-ebook/dp/B006T5JNGM

Beat Sugar Addiction Now!: The Cutting-Edge Program That Cures Your Type of Sugar Addiction
http://www.amazon.com/Beat-Sugar-Addiction-Now-ebook/dp/B004MME0OE

Beating Sugar Addiction For Dummies
http://www.amazon.com/Beating-Addiction-Dummies-Fitness-ebook/dp/B00CWZ9FEI

www.ingramcontent.com/pod-product-compliance
Lightning Source LLC
Chambersburg PA
CBHW071352310526
45750CB00018B/1424